HOW TO
BUILD
MUSCLE

CHRIS JANKE-BUENO

WHERE ARE THE EXERCISES?

This book is the first step in the My Core Balance strength program. It includes the eight foundational concepts.

The exercise portion of the program is available in video format, at *www.MyCoreBalance.com/muscle*.

CONTENTS

ACKNOWLEDGMENTS

The views I hold about strength training and muscle building have been largely formed by men who lived 100 years ago. Their common sense approach appeals to me far more than the "latest research" that has been performed in a lab. I find it far more valuable to immerse myself in the strategies of people who have walked their talk, and achieved results similar to those that I want to achieve, before bodybuilders started using steroids.

I'd like to also acknowledge Mike Dillinger for the insight that modern readers would appreciate a shorter book that is easy to consume. I like the idea of these micro-books. Thanks Mike.

CHAPTER 1
REAL MUSCLE vs "THE PUMP"

A few years ago, I had an experience that changed the way I view strength and muscle. It was enough to change my mind about the purpose of lifting weights.

I met a man named James who was in his late 50s, and I was immediately aware of his big arms and thick neck. I said something like, "oh where do you workout?" His response absolutely shocked me.

"It's been a while." In my mind I was thinking that a while was maybe a month. He continued, "yeah, I haven't lifted since high school."

My head exploded! What?!?

It had been nearly 40 years since this man had touched a weight, and he was still muscled as if he had worked out last week.

This stood in direct contrast to my experience. For example, my wife will occasionally comment about my appearance. Usually, if I just lifted weights earlier in the day, she'd say something like, "you look strong."

On the other hand, if it had been a while since my last workout, she could tell. And often would tell me that I look like I lost muscle.

How is it that this 60-year-old man still looks like he is strong even though he hasn't lifted a weight in decades? On the other hand, I "deflate" after just a few days of not lifting.

I had so many questions. Are there different types of muscle gain? Am I doing something wrong? Have I been doing the wrong thing for 25 years? Am I just spinning my wheels with my workouts?

Whatever this guy knew, I wanted to know. Whatever he did, I wanted to do.

Fast forward a few months...

Uncovering articles and books about building real strength became my obsession. I read books from early 20th century bodybuilders. These strong men lifted weights and developed amazing muscles before the advent of steroids. I knew they could be trusted. But their advice... was... different...

At that time, there were so many things I was doing wrong according to the old time strongmen:

They said allow yourself a few days to recover... I was lifting every day.

Slowly and systematically add weight to the bar each workout if you can... I was doing tricks such as drop sets and supersets, and trying to "feel the burn." Not caring about the weight on the bar.

They said do just a handful of full body compound movements… I was doing 30 to 40 sets of isolation movements for the arms because that's what I wanted to get bigger.

They said that it's not necessary to "train to failure." In fact, sometimes it is counterproductive… I was training to failure almost every time I picked up a weight, thinking that if I didn't train to failure then I wasn't actually accomplishing anything.

They said that the stronger you get, the more structural integrity you *should* have, and the less likely you are to get injured… For me, it seemed like I injured myself each time I went in the weight room. I remember in college not being able to walk after a weightlifting session.

Fast forward a few more months…

I began my experiment. I created a very

simple and systematic program, with the number one goal of building strength (by adding more weight to the bar when my body was able to). I took more rest days, some weeks only lifting one time. This is completely opposite from my six day per week "split routine" that I used to do.

I started to care less about my appearance and more about my strength. The irony is that as I began to care about aesthetics less and less, my results began to astound me and others.

I remember the first time it really hit me how incredible this new program was. My wife commented about how muscular I looked that day, and assumed that I had just finished my workout. I had that "pump." But that wasn't the pump. That was actually muscle. I hadn't worked out in six days! Yeah I still looked as if I had just finished a workout. My arms were getting bigger, my chest, back, and legs were getting bigger. My waist was getting smaller, so although I was actually gaining weight I had many people ask me if I was losing weight because they saw my waist line going down.

What a complete blast in the face. I felt like I was discovering a lost treasure chest, only the treasure was buried right in front of my nose the whole time.

What's the *actual* difference between "the pump" and real muscle?

To an outsider, lifting weights is lifting weights. There may not be any special distinction in your mind between me and James.

But the difference in result is astounding. Think of how he could maintain his muscular look for 40 years without lifting weights, and I would appear to lose muscle after just a few days of not lifting.

Why does this happen?

The main reason is that there are two types of muscle growth. I don't want to get too technical, so I will try to keep this simple.

The type of muscle growth that I used to do is called sarcoplasmic hypertrophy. "Hypertrophy" simply refers to the process of muscle growth. Sarcoplasmic refers to the sarcoplasm within the muscle. Sarcoplasm is basically water. When you workout, your body preferentially sends blood to the muscles, because that is the area that needs more nutrients. Because of this, the muscles appeal appear to swell during exercise. That swelling is called the pump, and the pump lasts for a day or two after. But it soon fades.

The other type of muscle growth is called myofibrillar hypertrophy. Again, hypertrophy just means muscle growth. Myofibrillar refers to the fibers, and the actual muscle fibers that are growing in size because of increased demands placed upon them.

Simply put, sarcoplasmic hypertrophy is the appearance of strength, whereas myofibrillar hypertrophy is *actual* strength (and you still *look* strong too).

I decided then and there that I did not

want to simply *appear* strong, I wanted to *be* strong.

When training the pump, my visits to the weight room looked more like magic tricks. I was trying to pull the wool over my own eyes. I did all the classic magic tricks, changing the work out every week, drop sets, supersets, etc. nothing produced long-term muscle growth. Just the appearance of muscle.

This is not all about aesthetics. At least for me it's not. But if it is for you, there's good news. You would look better if you follow this program than you will if you just pump the muscles. The form follows the function of a muscle.

If you focus on specific muscles, you are missing the boat. In reality, we train the body as one whole unit. If you isolate the body into its specific parts too much, then not only will you be structurally weaker, but you won't look as good either because you will not have the natural symmetry that is associated with full body strength.

This is about creating real, usable strength, that benefits you during your actual life.

When you need to get your luggage into the overhead compartment, you won't need to ask for help.

When your child jumps on your back, he won't knock you over.

You won't worry about parking far away from the grocery store. In fact, you won't even take the cart from the store to the car. You'll take the bags out and carry them yourself!

Are you convinced? Do you want to have muscles that last? Real muscles? If so, keep reading.

CHAPTER 2
PROGRESSIVE OVERLOAD

Have you heard the story of the man who bought a baby cow? He carried this calf up a hill every day, and as the calf got bigger, he got stronger.

Progression is the first concept that I talk about in this book because I believe it is the most important. When somebody asks me, "what workout should I be doing?" My response is "well, what are you doing right now?" I listen carefully to their answers and I try to figure out what the next logical step will be.

When you're thinking about your fitness goals, all you need to know is where you are and what the next step is. Just. One.

Step.

The story of the man and the cow is a great analogy for building strength. It is exactly how the process works. It's baby steps all the way up the hill. It's so vitally important that you start small. Gradually, you will be able to progress. Whether that progression entails adding weight to the bar each workout, being able to stay on a machine for more time, or even simply getting better at the form of an exercise, your body has no choice but to adapt as you start getting stronger.

Your muscles will not get stronger unless they have to. The only way to force a muscle to be stronger is to go slightly outside of your comfort zone, allow yourself to recover, and then do it again. When you workout the next time, your "comfort zone" is slightly expanded.

When you're assessing your progress, the number one question you can ask yourself is, "am I better than yesterday? Better than last week? Last month?"

Make self-improvement your number one goal. Progress constantly, and you will always be getting closer to your final destination.

CHAPTER 3
CONSISTENCY

About one year ago I tried an experiment. Instead of setting a big goal about how much weight I wanted to lift or what I wanted to look like, I set an incredibly small goal. My goal was to show up to the gym every single day.

I structured my goal so it was achievable. It's not possible to do intense workouts everyday, especially when you're first starting to get in shape. My goal was winnable: just show up.

Several days I remember waking up in a horrible mood, body aching from the day before, and generally just not wanting to exercise. On those days I still laced up my shoes and drove to the gym. One day I just sat in the steam room for 5 minutes, took a shower, and left. Another day I went to an empty group exercise room and took a nap.

Despite the non-workouts, those days were victories for me. I maintained my momentum. Momentum is the key ingredient to get healthy and fit. Momentum turns small daily workouts into lifelong health. Momentum makes it easy to wake up in the morning. Negative momentum can even turn missed workouts into body fat.

I have four children. Each time a new baby is born, there are sleepless nights. But this is not a free pass to skip my gym time. By making my goal super achievable, just going after perfect attendance, I can create momentum toward my ultimate fitness goals.

From here on, adopt this as your central philosophy. The only time you miss a workout is if there is a birth, death, or an emergency that you would have to call

9-1-1. That's it. Otherwise we are lifting. We are running. We are stretching. And on those really "bad" days, we are simply just showing up.

If the pope is coming to town and you want to meet him, great. Workout first.

If you couldn't sleep all night because the dog next-door was barking, sorry to hear that. Go to the gym.

If you have to pick up the kids from school during your normal gym time, schedule the gym for another time. Go to the gym. If your kids are old enough, bring them with you.

If you are sick, go on a light walk instead. Don't get everyone at the gym sick too. But do something.

If you're tired, go to the gym and just sit in the sauna. Just show up. Do something.

I think you see the common theme here. There's no real reason to skip the gym.

In this book, I'm going to give you the exact workouts that I am personally doing at this point in my life. I'm 39 years old, and I can honestly say that I am in the best shape of my life. When I was in high school, I could run faster and farther, but I had back pain. When I was in my early 20s I could dunk a basketball, but I wasn't very strong. In my late 20s, I had the back pain under control, but was very underweight, lacking strength and muscle. Now, I have put it all together into an inclusive program.

As great as these exercises are, they are nothing without consistency. A consistent workout program is more valuable than an inconsistent workout program. Once you develop consistency, then you can start exercising with more intensity. Consistency comes first, and then intensity is the natural byproduct of that consistency.

Consistency is one of the first "muscles" you need to train. Once you have mastered the art of consistency, you will see how easy it is to make subtle changes that will make drastic improvements toward your fitness goals. Success in fitness is absolutely impossible without being consistent.

CHAPTER 4
HAVE A LONG-TERM VISION

This might sound like a weird question, but do you think you will be alive in a year? Hopefully the answer is yes. Now another question. If you are going to be alive anyway, why not give the "future you" a present? Let's give you of the future the gift of good health.

When undergoing a big body transformation, you need to think in terms of quarters and years, not days and weeks. In mid November 2018, I woke up in the middle of the night with an awareness. I realized that today is my half birthday. I was 38½. 18 months until 40.

What do I want to look and feel like on that 40th birthday? That's the kind of long range planning I'm talking about.

Later on in the book you will get a chance to set your goals for the quarter. Three months is a great amount of time relating to fitness because it's long enough where you can actually get a lot of work done and make some good changes, yet it's short enough to stay motivated.

Beyond those 90 days, you also need a bigger vision that will drive you forward. This vision needs to include what you plan to accomplish, and also why you want to accomplish it. The key is that the "why" needs to be compelling to you. It needs to be something that you find valuable and beneficial. You should be able to integrate this into the rest of your life's goals. Make sure you see the big picture.

So although we will be working in terms of a 90-day goal in this book, make sure these 90 days fit into a larger, more compelling vision for your fitness and your life.

What do you want? Can you imagine your life in one year? Two? Three? Three years is long enough to go from dozens (or hundreds!) of pounds overweight to being a pillar of health. Even one year is enough time to create a complete 180-degree transformation. But you have to have a vision. You have to know where you're going.

Barring some birth defect, genetic abnormality, or big accident, anybody can achieve pretty much any fitness goals that they set their mind to. It's not easy, and there will be challenging workouts. There will also be times when you lose motivation. Having a clear and compelling big picture vision is how you navigate through that.

Take a little bit of time and let your imagination run wild. If you could have the body of your dreams, what would it look and feel like?

Download a SMART Goals worksheet at www.MyCoreBalance.com/muscle, and spend some good quality time daydreaming, working out what you want to achieve in your head. Once it's in your head and heart, you can achieve it in your life.

CHAPTER 5
KEEP IT SIMPLE AND FUN

We've done some serious goal setting and soul-searching so far, which can sometimes make people get too serious. Remember, it's also very important to keep it fun.

As a kid, I always considered recess and lunch to be my favorite school activities. I would imagine that most of the kids would agree with that, that they would rather be out on the playground than sitting in a classroom listening to the teacher.

But as an adult, I'm surprised at how many people don't enjoy exercise. They don't consider their workout to be their break to recharge and feel good again. It's something to dread and "get through" so you can move on to the rest of your life.

As much as I love health and fitness, I must blame the fitness industry for this dread. The only reason why somebody wouldn't like exercise is because he thinks it should be hard, boring, and tedious. When we realize that exercise should be fun, exhilarating, and uplifting, then we will have a natural and intrinsic desire to move more.

If you are just beginning your fitness journey, it's vitally important that you do something that energizes you. You should do something that you enjoy. Even if that means you just go on a walk in nature, or play with your kids, investing in the fun of exercise is important.

If you asked your doctor how much time you need to spend every day exercising, she will most likely give you generic medical advice, which is 45 minutes five days per week or something like that.

But if you haven't been doing anything up until now, 45 minutes is a long time! So instead of shooting for a big arbitrary goal, just aim for progress. If you have not been working out, workout for five minutes. If you're already doing 20 minutes, try 25. If you've already been working out for an hour twice per week, make it three times per week.

Simple, right? Keep it simple, keep it doable, and progress is assured.

This coincides with the earlier principle of progression. It doesn't have to be complicated, you just need to know where you are and take the next step.

Simplicity works!

Over the past 12 months, I've gained more than 15 pounds of muscle. During this time, I've done only two workouts, Workout A and Workout B. I've lifted an average of just two days per week. Currently, I have dropped my lifting down to just **ONCE PER WEEK**, and results have actually improved.

I could not have made these strides doing a traditional bodybuilding plan (5 days per week, splitting the body into parts), or using gimmicks like drop sets, supersets, etc.

CHAPTER 6
MASTER FORM FIRST,
THEN WORK HARD

As a beginner, your main goal is to improve your form. Your mechanics need to be spot on. So feel free to take 3 to 9 months just to work on your technique. Use a wooden closet rod instead of an actual weight. Really make sure you dial it in.

Don't do weighted squats, do bodyweight squats. Don't do weighted windmills, do side to side windmill motion without weight. Do Bench Press with a closet rod instead of a barbell.

Start light! Start extremely light! Start with a weight so light that you could do 1,000 repetitions in a row. You will have plenty of time to progress. In the meantime, fix muscle imbalances, work on form, try to really understand what you're doing at a deep level.

Once you've progressed past the beginner phase, begin to progress by adding weight. Always make sure your **FORM** stays good, you **FEEL** the right muscles, and your **SPEED** is slow and controlled.

Although these concepts are extremely simple, getting strong is not easy. There's plenty of hard work. After you pass the beginning stages, the weights start to get heavy.

Now you've past the learning phase, so it's time to really work. Here's a great rule to think about. If you look at the programs later in the book, you may think that they don't look so complicated. They're not. Doing a basic exercise with a heavy weight (heavy for you, not compared to somebody else). All of a sudden you make the simplest exercise very challenging.

After you finish a set of any challenging exercise, if you feel like you can go directly into the next set, you are not working even close to as hard as we need to to build muscle. After a set, you should need to rest for at least 30 seconds. *At least*! Sometimes I have to rest for several minutes before I feel like I have the strength to do another set. You really need to push yourself.

Everything else always applies to keep you safe, such as good form, feeling the right muscle, slow and controlled cadence... Focus on all those things and then work hard!

I cannot overstate this point. If you are not making progress, it's probably because you're not working hard enough. And if you are not making progress, but you think you are working hard enough, then you don't really know what hard work is.

I would not call myself an "in-your-face" personal trainer. I am more chill and laid-back. But make no mistake about it, when I get into the gym, I work hard. And you should too.

CHAPTER 7
PRACTICAL NUTRITION

I call this "Plus One Habit Creation," where you gradually add one habit until mastered. It's a very simple way to go from 0% to 100% without skipping any steps.

Here's how to do it:

Work on one task at a time. First, start with #1. Once you've mastered that for a week or so, keep it as a habit and add #2. Progress through the list until you've systematically added all 7 habits.

With nutrition, follow this list. The full, detailed explanation of the following seven steps is available in my other book **_"Help! My Diet Sucks!"_**

Seven simple nutrition steps:

1. Cut all beverages except water, drink ½ to 1 gallon of water per day.
2. Drink a green fruit / vegetable smoothie daily.
3. Cut packaged snacks, replace with fruits and vegetables.
4. Cut fried food, hydrogenated oils, and trans fats. And add healthy fats.
5. Cut out processed protein, and add natural protein.
6. Convert starchy carbs to green carbs.
7. Practice perfect proportions (divide your plate equally between protein, carbs, fat, and greens).

There are a bazillion diets out there, and I'm sure a lot of them are good. (Of course, a lot of them are bad also). I'm less concerned about following some sort of "diet," and more concerned about you making food choices that are easy to implement in your life and sticking to those so that you feel good about your decisions. Keep it simple.

CHAPTER 8
REST AND RECOVERY

I got my first taste of weightlifting when I was 14 years old. My dad and I got memberships to the local YMCA and would visit there three days a week to lift. Looking back, I realize how great of a bonding experience this was, and how much I learned.

My dad is one of those men similar to James that I talked about earlier in the book. He played football in high school, and he wrestled in high school and college. My dad's shoulders and back were thick because he lifted weights when he was younger.

When I was 14 years old, my dad was 51. As far as I know he hadn't lifted since high school, yet here he was with more muscle than me. Despite being a know-it-all teenager, I knew he had much to teach me. And I listened when he spoke.

One day I was getting frustrated with my slow progress. And trying to think of a shortcut, I mentioned that what we should do is design a machine that stimulates the muscles so we could activate them all night while we were sleeping. What my dad said in response has stayed with me for the last 25 years.

"You don't grow muscle while you're lifting weights. You grow muscle while you sleep." That's all he needed to say for me to change my mind.

10 years later I became a personal trainer, and I learned about the mechanisms of recovery. What is far more of a determining factor as to whether somebody is going to gain a lot of muscle or not has more to do with their nutrition

and sleep patterns. The workout is one component of the bigger picture.

Somewhere during your training plan you will probably lose patience like I did. This will probably come somewhere between month 6 and 12. You've been doing the plan long enough to get results, yet not long enough to experience huge results.

When this time comes, and you are tempted to shortcut the process, remember that there are no shortcuts. Do everything right, and in a matter of quarters or years you will have your results.

If we look at this a little closer, we realize that the weights actually make us weaker. Think about it, at the end of your workout you are weaker than when you went in. What's the point of that? Why would you deliberately want to make yourself weaker? Well, the answer is because of that adaptation that happens within your body because of the workout.

Don't overdo it. Don't overdo it. And

again... ***DO NOT OVERDO IT!***

So many people become addicted to the actual *process* of exercise. Yes, it's true, exercise is an end in itself (it can be fun), but it's also a means to an end. It's important to remember what your goals are. By lifting weights every day, you neglect the restful aspect of a weight training routine and run the serious and probable risk of over-training.

Remember the purpose of exercise. We want to exercise in order to build up, not break down. We want more structural integrity, not less. We want to feel better, not worse. We are working out for our future self, and don't want to be injured when we're 70.

CHAPTER 9
THE WORKOUTS

The simple concepts that you just read are enough to get you in the right frame of mind to build muscle. Now it's time to move!

The specific workouts are available in video format, at *www.MyCoreBalance.com/muscle.*

Visit that page now to get started.

Dear Reader,

Although the concepts are simple, strength training is not easy. It takes coordination, discipline, and the ability to plan your schedule on a day-to-day practical level, and then follow through with that plan.

This book fits into a larger system, one that I have created over the past 15 years.

The foundation of that system is a healthy, pain-free back and proper nutrition.

I recommend using my other two books to create that foundation. Be sure to check out ***Help! I threw Out My Back!*** and ***Help! My Diet Sucks!*** Both titles are available in paperback on Amazon. Also visit www.MyCoreBalance.com for more programs.

Use this book as a resource for years to come. And if you stumble upon anything that the book does not address, text your questions to me at 408–883–4442.

Your friend in Health,

www.ingramcontent.com/pod-product-compliance
Lightning Source LLC
Chambersburg PA
CBHW061739250726
48657CB00002B/1007